Keto Kickstart

Table of Contents

Disclaimer

Copyright © 2020

All Rights Reserved.

This book is not written by a medical doctor and does not provide cures for any diseases. Please consult a professional doctor if you are sick.

Introduction

The ketogenic diet is among the most popular diets today due to its simplicity. Most people follow the ketogenic diet because it is famous, or because they have heard about the amazing benefits it offers.

Research shows that the ketogenic diet helps to reduce weight, reset your metabolism, improve your health and increase your energy. This book provides detailed information on the ketogenic diet and its benefits. You will learn about the various types of food you can and cannot eat when you follow the diet, and learn how your body works when you reduce your carbohydrate intake. The book also talks about the science behind the diet, and how it affects your hormones and metabolism.

When the ketogenic diet became popular, many questions and myths around this diet came into existence. This book will clear those common myths and beliefs about the diet. Many people find it difficult to follow the ketogenic diet, or any diet for that matter since it is hard for them to adhere to the rules. The diet is quite simple to follow, but many people are not able to sustain because they give into their cravings.

If you have recently switched to the ketogenic diet and find it difficult to maintain, then your first focus should be on consuming the right foods. The book has some tips, which you can use to make it easier for you to ease into your diet and stick to. Some people make mistakes when they follow the diet, and that is where this book will help them, as the information given in this book will ensure you avoid making common mistakes that may throw you off balance from the diet.

Research shows that it is difficult for women to lose weight when compared to men. That can happen due to multiple reasons. However, it deters women from following and sticking to most diets because they do not see results immediately. This book provides information on why the ketogenic diet is good for women, and what they should do to tweak the diet to suit their body.

If you are new to the diet, then you can use the 15-day meal plan at the end of the book. The meals in the plan are simple to make. It is important to note that you cannot lose weight only by following a diet, and the ketogenic diet is no different. You also need to exercise regularly, sleep well and reduce stress levels.

So without any further ado, let us get started and learn more about the keto diet.

Thank you once again for choosing this book. I hope you get all the information about the ketogenic diet and get started.

Part One: What is the Ketogenic Diet, the Science Behind the Diet and Myths and Beliefs

An Introduction to the Ketogenic Diet

The ketogenic diet may seem overwhelming at first. However, when you follow the diet, you will realize it isn't as difficult as you perceived it to be. The more you learn about this diet, the more you realize it is simple and easy to follow. Even if you are on a budget or feel like the keto diet has too many restrictions, there are different methods and tips you can use to keep the diet simple. Before we get into that, let us first learn what the keto diet is.

What is the Ketogenic diet?

The primary purpose of the keto diet is to shift your body into the state of ketosis, so it uses fats as the main source of energy instead of carbohydrates. When your body shifts into this state, it helps you lose weight, prevent brain fog and offers a lot of other benefits. To induce ketosis, you must:

- Drastically reduce your carbohydrate intake, so your body resorts to using the fat reserves to produce energy.
- Follow a low-carb diet while still providing your body with the required macronutrient intake

You can easily do this by following the keto diet. The dietary requirements of macronutrients are divided as follows:

- 5% – 10% carbohydrates

- 55% - 60% fats

- 30% - 35% protein

If you consume 2000 Calories a day, your carbohydrate intake should amount to only 10 – 25 grams. When you reduce your carbohydrate intake, your body begins to burn fat reserves to produce energy. We will learn more about this later in the book.

What are Ketones?

When you reduce your carbohydrate intake, your body does not have enough glucose to produce energy, and it looks for alternate energy sources. Your liver breaks the fat down to provide your body with energy. It is during this chemical process, that your liver forms ketone bodies. These bodies shift the body into the metabolic state known as ketosis. This metabolic state helps you lose weight.

Tips to maintain ketosis

This section leaves you with some tips to help you maintain ketosis.

Restricting carbohydrates

As mentioned in the previous section, you need to reduce your carbohydrate intake to 10 – 25 grams per day. Since most food groups contain carbohydrates, it is best to choose the ones with fewer carbs. When you reduce your carbohydrate intake, your body automatically shifts into ketosis to find alternate energy sources.

Restricting protein

When you limit your protein consumption to 30% of your daily calorie intake, you can maintain ketosis. If you consume too much protein, your body learns to break the macronutrient into glucose, which shifts your body out of ketosis. Therefore, you should learn to maintain your protein intake.

Enough fats

When you eat saturated, healthy fat, it becomes easier to control your hunger. If you are hungry all the time, increase your fat and not your carbohydrate intake. This way you can ensure that your body does not switch out of ketosis.

Avoid snacking

Do not eat when you are not hungry, and this means you should avoid untimely snacking too. Emotional eating or eating just for fun because you cannot resist food slows down the process of ketosis, thereby decreasing your chances of weight loss.

Sleep enough

People who are sleep deprived find it extremely difficult to get into ketosis, which makes it harder for them to lose weight. Sleep deprivation can cause the stress hormone to rise, which in-turn increases your blood-sugar levels and slows down ketosis. So, make sure you sleep enough if you follow the keto diet.

Is Keto a Healthier Way to Live?

You should avoid diets that create a disconnect between your body's basic instincts about food. Take yo-yo dieting for example. People following fad diets find themselves oscillating between being "up to the mark" and then suddenly "falling off the wagon" too often. Keto, on the other hand, is a way of life more than a diet. This diet does not restrict your caloric intake and allows you to eat healthy meals. You can eat as much food as you want, as long as you follow the plan. It also ensures that your body is never low on nutrition, thereby keeping you energized, and in a positive mood throughout the day. This is a good enough reason to adopt the ketogenic diet as a regular dietary pattern.

Science Behind the Ketogenic Diet

Metabolism and Ketogenic Diet

Metabolism is one of the most important aspects to consider when you follow any diet or weight loss program. When you consume enough carbohydrates, there is enough glucose in your body to produce energy. Since your body does not require fat to produce energy, it will save the excess fat as a reserve.

Balanced diets contain the right amount of carbohydrates, fats and proteins. When there is a carbohydrate deficit, your body uses the carbohydrate reserves to produce energy. Once these reserves deplete, it looks for an alternative energy source. It begins to target the fat reserves in your body to produce energy. When your body burns fatty acids, it produces ketones. These ketones are neither fat nor carbohydrates, but your body uses them as energy. When you create a carbohydrate deficit, your body shifts into ketosis, and uses the fat reserves to produce energy.

During ketosis, your body releases ketones into the blood stream. This reduces the production of glucose in your body thereby increasing the usage of already present glucose. Your body begins to use any excess fat to provide you with the energy you need.

Hormones and the Ketogenic Diet

Your hormones maintain the functioning of your body, and the food you eat has a significant impact on your body. Your body releases certain hormones depending on the food you consume.

As mentioned earlier, your body needs to adapt to the changes in your diet when you follow the ketogenic diet. Since you drastically reduce your carbohydrate intake, the insulin and glucagon levels in your body drop. Insulin is a hormone that helps to move the nutrients to your blood steam and store them. It also controls the blood sugar levels. Insulin stores glucose released during digestion in the form of glycogen. The hormone Glucagon helps to break glycogen down to provide your body with the right amounts of glucose. This helps to reduce blood sugar level.

When you stop consuming a large amount of carbohydrates, the insulin levels decrease in your body while the glucagon levels increase. This ensures that your body burns the fat cells to produce enough energy to help you sustain throughout the day. The liver burns the excess fat in your body, and this chemical reaction produces ketones. When the ketones move into your bloodstream, your body shifts into ketosis. This metabolic state affects many hormones and can cause some fluctuation in the production of cortisol, estrogen and insulin.

Exercise and the ketogenic diet

Most people do not like to exercise, but want to lose weight quickly. They try many fad diets to lose weight, but one of the best ways to lose weight is by exercising. When you follow the ketogenic diet, the best time to workout is in the morning before breakfast, since you give your body sufficient time to burn the food you ate the previous night, it will turn to the fat reserves to produce energy. Some people choose to work out in the evening or night, and that is okay too.

You need to ensure you exercise regularly and get at least two or three high intensity workouts every week. When you exercise your muscles every day, you ensure that your body has lesser calories to burn. It is only for this reason that most athletes eat more proteins and fewer carbohydrates. Athletes try to jump start the ketosis process to strengthen their body. This metabolic state helps to increase the lean muscle mass in the body.

Myths and Beliefs

Ever since the diet gained popularity, there are many myths and misconceptions around the diet. This chapter debunks some myths of the diet.

Your Body Shifts into the Ketoacidosis State

As mentioned earlier, ketosis burns excess fat in the body. When you follow the ketogenic diet, your body shifts into ketosis where it uses fat to produce energy. During the process of ketosis, it breaks the fat molecules to produce energy, and the by-product of this reaction are the ketone bodies. This process is different from diabetic ketoacidosis, which is a complication of diabetes. This complication occurs when your body does not produce enough insulin, but the ketone levels increase.

You Can Switch Between a Keto and a Normal Diet

The reality is that you will gain the weight you lost if you switch between the ketogenic diet and a normal diet. Most people do not understand the ketogenic diet, and they jump into it without learning more about how it works. They tend to follow the diet for a couple of days, and then go back to eating the usual number of carbohydrates the following day. You will not produce ketones and gain the benefits of this diet if you continue to behave this way.

Everybody Needs the Same Number of Carbs

Your carbohydrate intake depends on your personal health. When you follow a low-carb diet, you do not realize how low in carbohydrates the diet actually is. Most people who follow the ketogenic diet restrict their carbohydrate intake to 20-25 grams each day. They try to minimize their carb intake, so their body switches into ketosis easily. You can consume more carbohydrates depending on how active you are and what stage of ketosis you are in. Consult a dietician or nutritionist to calculate your requirements.

You Can Eat as Much Butter and Bacon as You Want

When you follow the ketogenic diet, you need to increase your intake of fats, but this does not mean you increase your intake of saturated fat. Do not eat a plate of bacon in the morning for breakfast. The healthiest way to increase your fat intake is to limit the consumption of saturated fat, like sausage and bacon and instead increase your intake of olive oil, avocado oil, flaxseeds nuts and other good fats. We will look at the different foods you can and cannot eat in the following chapter.

Avoid All Fruit and Vegetables Since they are High in Carbs

One major side effect of the keto diet is constipation, and to avoid this side effect you need to increase your fiber intake. Fruit and vegetables are good sources of carbohydrates, but this does not mean you stop eating them all. Unprocessed and whole foods are good sources of vitamins, minerals, fiber and antioxidants. Consume non-starchy vegetables such as cauliflower, zucchini, broccoli, cucumber and peppers. You can also consume low-carb fruit such as blueberries, raspberries, melons and strawberries. The next chapter lists the different foods you can and cannot consume when you follow the keto diet. Always consult this list before you prepare a meal.

You Should Consume More Protein

The ketogenic diet is a low-carb diet, but it is very different from other low carb diets, such as the Atkins Diet. You can consume a bowl of smoked salmon and eggs for breakfast and eat steak for dinner, but you should consume protein in moderation. As mentioned earlier, when you consume excess protein, your body converts it to glucose thereby increasing the blood sugar levels that will take your body out of ketosis. The number of ketone bodies in your blood also increases when your body burns more amino acids. This leads to ketoacidosis, which can harm your bones. If you do not know how much protein you need to consume, speak to your dietician or nutritionist about the same. Identify the macro breakdown that works for your body.

This Diet is the Best Way to Lose Weight

The keto diet is not a one-stop solution. It does not work for everybody, just like every other diet. A friend of yours may have lost a lot of weight when he followed the ketogenic diet, but this does not mean the diet will work in the same manner for you. You need to ensure you do adequate exercise and maintain an active lifestyle along with the diet for best results.

Keto is Not a Long-Term Weight Loss Solution

Studies show that the ketogenic diet is ideal to manage weight in the long-term. Research also shows that people who follow the ketogenic diet lost more weight when compared to people who followed a low-fat diet.

Keto Diet Causes a Lack of Sleep

There is no foundation for this myth; rather people who consume low-carb diets sleep better. Research shows that people who follow the ketogenic diet sleep better than those who follow other low-fat diets.

Keto Leads to Acne

Research shows that carbohydrates cause acne, and low-carb and low-glycemic diets reduced breakouts.

Food to Eat and Avoid

In this chapter, we will look at what foods you should consume and which ones to keep at bay while following the ketogenic diet.

Food to Eat

Cruciferous Vegetables

Cruciferous vegetables are rich in fiber, antioxidants, vitamins and minerals, but are low in carbohydrates. They are also rich in Vitamins A and K and sulforaphane. Your body produces the latter when you chew or crush cruciferous vegetables. When your body digests this compound, it activates a protective shield around cells to prevent oxidation. This shield decreases the risk of cancer and heart diseases and improves cognitive function. If you want to remain in ketosis, avoid the consumption of starchy vegetables, and increase your consumption of starchy vegetables.

High Fat Dairy

High-fat dairy contains high-quality protein, conjugated linoleic acid, vitamins and minerals. Your body needs the combination of these nutrients to improve and maintain body functions and strength as you age. A study conducted to understand the effect of high-fat dairy on aging people concluded that the consumption of seven to ten ounces of ricotta cheese increased muscle strength and mass in older participants. This means you do not have to reduce your consumption of cream, butter and cheese. Since high-fat dairy contains fewer carbohydrates, include a reasonable amount of any dairy product in every meal.

Avocado

Increase your intake of avocados when you follow the ketogenic diet, especially if you have recently started the diet. This fruit is rich in several minerals and vitamins, like potassium. When you increase your potassium intake, you can reduce the symptoms of keto flu. These symptoms include constant headaches, fatigue, feeling feverish. Avocados are also known to improve triglyceride and cholesterol levels, and you can use avocado oil instead if you do not like the fruit. Avocado oil contains monosaturated fat, which helps to improve cholesterol levels in the body.

Berries

Most fruit are rich in carbohydrates and sugar, and hence cannot be consumed on the ketogenic diet. Berries and some other fruit, however, are an exception. You can choose from different types of berries, such as strawberries, blueberries and blackberries, and each type contains different forms of anthocyanins. These compounds give berries their color and have anti-inflammatory effects on the body. Research shows that wild blueberries prevent inflammation in the brain and improve memory as you age. That said, you should consume moderate quantities of berries to maintain your carbohydrate and sugar intake.

Olive oil and olives

Olives and virgin olive oil contain many health-promoting compounds and oleocanthal, a phenolic compound. Research shows that both olives and olive oil have anti-inflammatory properties similar to that of ibuprofen. That said, you must only consume the required amount of olive oil to ensure you do not consume more than the required quantity of fat.

Coconut oil

Coconut oil is known to help the body to shift easily into the state of ketosis. It is for this reason some people drink a cup of coffee every morning with coconut oil, also known as bullet coffee. Coconut oil is rich in medium chain triglycerides (MCT), and your body can absorb this fat easily, and move it to the liver. Your body either stores the fat or burns it depending on your carbohydrate intake. Coconut oil has four forms of MCTs, but most of the fat in coconut oil is found in the form of lauric acid. Studies show that fat sources with a higher concentration of lauric acid ensure you stay in ketosis longer than other forms of MCTs. You can also use MCTs to induce the state of ketosis in children with epilepsy without reducing their intake of carbohydrates. When you add coconut oil to your diet, add it slowly to minimize any side effects like diarrhea and stomach cramps. Start with half a teaspoon per day and slowly work up to two teaspoons over the course of one week.

Meat, Seafood and Poultry

Poultry, seafood and meat are food groups rich in protein. These foods also contain essential vitamins and minerals, like Vitamin B12, which is an essential nutrient since it is a highly absorbable form of creatine, iron, carnosine, DHA and taurine. Poultry and fresh meat are packed with several other vitamins and minerals. Always consume 100% grass-fed meat and pasture-raised poultry to ensure you obtain the required levels of nutrients. These products contain more antioxidants when compared to grain-fed meat products. The same can be said about shellfish, but it is important to understand number of carbohydrates present in different types of fish. Most people following the ketogenic diet often eat more protein since they like meat and seafood. It is important to spread the amount of protein consumed between different meals to maintain ketone levels.

Eggs

Eggs are considered as one of the most versatile and healthiest foods. Many experts suggest that eggs are a type of 'superfood.' The thirteen essential minerals and vitamins, and the antioxidants that protect the eye like zeaxanthin and lutein are found in eggs. The yolk is also the best source of choline, which is a methyl donor and an essential nutrient involved in multiple physiological processes.

Egg yolks contain high levels of cholesterol, however; the cholesterol levels in your body do not fluctuate when you eat eggs. Research shows that eggs can modify the shape of LDL cholesterol to reduce the risk of any heart disease. The consumption of eggs keeps the levels of blood sugar stable and also satiates your hunger. This helps you decrease your caloric intake automatically which shows that eggs can help you lose weight easily. One large egg only contains one gram of carbs and close to 6 grams of protein, which makes this dish the perfect keto-friendly health food.

Dark Chocolate

Dark chocolate, unlike other forms of chocolate, is good for your health and contains flavonol, which reduces the risk of heart disease, insulin resistance and blood pressure. Cocoa, also known as superfruit, contains the same number of antioxidants as any other keto-friendly fruit. However, you can't eat as much dark chocolate when you follow the ketogenic diet. Dark chocolate is also rich in carbohydrates, and when you consume too much chocolate, your body automatically shifts out of ketosis. When you buy any cocoa product or chocolate, read the label and ensure there are no added sugars. Also look at the number of carbs per serving of the chocolate.

Foods to Avoid

Starches and Grains

Most people eat bread in some form every day. It is convenient to run to the grocery store and pick up a sandwich. Bread is one food group that goes with every meal, and people avoid the ketogenic diet when they are asked to give up bread. Grains cause a lot of problems to the body. Recently, people have begun to switch to gluten-free food. When you cut grains out from your diet, you cut out tons of carbohydrates. You do not need to fret since people following the keto diet are innovative and if they want to eat bread, they are going to find some way to do that. The same can be said for rice. If you want to eat rise, make yourself some cauliflower rice.

Alcohol

Avoid alcohol regardless of what type of diet you follow. Since you have to watch your carbohydrate intake when you follow the ketogenic diet, avoid the consumption of drinks rich in carbohydrates, including:

- Liqueurs

- Ciders
- Beer

You can drink the following in moderation:

- Gin
- Whiskey
- Scotch
- Tequila
- Vodka
- Rum
- Brandy
- Cognac

If you find yourself in a situation where you have to drink alcohol, try to get out of it.

Sugar

Most people enjoy fruit and candy and eat them as a snack. When you follow the ketogenic diet, you may need to give up on some fruit since they are rich in carbohydrates and sugar. This increases your carbohydrate intake and shifts your body out of ketosis. You must, therefore, control your intake of fruit and candy if you want to stay in ketosis. This does not mean you cannot eat any candy; you can instead gorge on fat bombs. However, be careful with the number of fat bombs you eat. You should avoid the following if you follow the ketogenic diet:

- Ice cream
- Fruit juices
- Pastries
- Cookies
- Sodas

If you love fruit, grab a bowl of berries when you crave sweets, but watch your consumption.

Benefits of the Ketogenic Diet

There is a lot of negativity that surrounds the ketogenic diet, and there are many misconceptions about the diet. This chapter sheds some light on the benefits of the diet. We will also look at some side effects of this diet. It is best to learn both the benefits and side effects, so you know what you are getting yourself into.

Reduced appetite

Most people find it hard to stick to their diets because they eat when they are bored and are often hungry because they avoid consuming too much food. The advantage with the ketogenic diet is that you remain energetic throughout the day since your body will burn fatty acids to produce energy. This will reduce your appetite drastically. Numerous studies show that people who follow a low-carb diet tend to eat fewer calories.

Loss of abdominal fat

People believe that they can lose fat only through exercise, and they work on exercises that target specific muscles in the body. What they tend to forget is that the different fat stored in the body is not the same. There are two types of fat in the body – the visceral fat and the subcutaneous fat. Visceral fat is found in the abdominal region, and this fat is dangerous since it will surround itself against the different organs. When you follow the ketogenic diet, your body will target the fat reserves to produce energy, and it will first target the visceral fat. When you lose fat in the abdomen, you can reduce the risk of heart diseases and Type II Diabetes.

Weight Loss

When on a diet, people often forget to consider the carbohydrates that they eat in every meal. Ketogenic diet is a low carbohydrate diet, which assists in the weight loss process. When you eat fewer carbohydrates, your body sheds excess water it stores, thereby reducing the levels of insulin in your body, which directly impact the levels of sodium in your body and induces weight loss. Research has confirmed that a low carbohydrate diet will help a person lose weight faster than many other diets.

Lower Blood Pressure

People who have high blood pressure are at a higher risk of developing heart diseases. Hypertension can also lead to kidney damage or failure, which is dangerous for the body. When you follow a low-carb diet, your blood pressure reduces thereby decreasing the risk of developing heart diseases.

Lower Blood Sugar Levels

When you lower your intake of carbohydrates, the blood glucose levels decrease. This helps to decrease the risk of developing Type II diabetes. If you have Type II diabetes, you should follow the ketogenic diet to manage and maintain the insulin levels in your body.

Your body breaks carbohydrates into smaller sugars in the digestive tract. These sugars enter the bloodstream and increase your blood sugar levels. Your body will then produce insulin, which will move the glucose from the bloodstream to different parts of the body. Insulin will indicate to the cells that they need to store the glucose in them or burn them to produce energy. When people are healthy, the insulin in their body helps to reduce the level of sugar in the blood, which will helps to protect us from any harm. Some people develop insulin resistance, which makes it difficult for the body to move the sugar from the bloodstream to the cells. This leads to Type II diabetes.

When you lower your intake of carbohydrates, your blood sugar levels do not fluctuate. This helps to reduce the risk of developing Type II diabetes.

Reduces the Symptoms of Metabolic Syndrome

Most people tend to have the metabolic syndrome and are blind to it. If you have any of the symptoms mentioned below, it is best if you switched to a low carbohydrate diet.

- High Levels of Blood Sugar
- Low levels of HDL
- Excess Visceral Fat
- Hypertension or high blood pressure
- High levels of Triglycerides

The ketogenic diet helps to reduce the symptoms mentioned thereby reducing the risk of heart diseases and diabetes.

There are certain organizations that have stated that low fat diets are better when compared to low carbohydrate diets since they cater to any metabolic issues that you may have. Research conducted on the diet says otherwise.

Side Effects

Like every other diet, the ketogenic diet also has significant effects on your body. That said, this diet is safer when compared to other diets. You should consider the effects of this diet on your body if you choose to follow it and find a way to minimize the symptoms. Based on the side effects mentioned below, you can make an informed decision before you start this diet.

Short term side effects

There are numerous short-term side effects obvious to the eye, when you initially start the diet. One of the most common effects is hypoglycemia. The symptoms of this side effect are:

1. Fatigue
2. Constant urination
3. Anxiety, irritability and confusion
4. Excessive thirst
5. Hunger
6. Sweating
7. Shakiness
8. Chills
9. Tachycardia

Some people also experience low-grade acidosis and constipation. The symptoms reduce over time if you continue with the diet since your body begins to adapt to these changes and will try to identify newer ways to source energy.

Alteration in the blood composition

Due to changes in the diet, your body also makes some changes to adapt to the reduced carbohydrate intake. As mentioned earlier, the ketogenic diet helps to lower blood sugar levels since you decrease your consumption of carbohydrates.

Research shows that people who follow this diet have higher levels of lipids and cholesterol (which is good cholesterol) than what is considered to be normal. More than 60% of the people following this diet had raised lipid levels and 30% had raised cholesterol levels.

If these changes are profound, they may affect you. Check your cholesterol levels and blood composition frequently to ensure you are eating well. For instance, the individual could substitute the saturated fats in his food with polyunsaturated fats.

Long Term Effects

When you follow this diet for a longer period, there are certain adverse effects that become more evident. These effects have a significant impact on your physical, mental and emotional health.

Kidney stones are a common complication that may occur in children and adults. Close to 5% of the people following the diet suffer from this complication. This is a complication that you can treat easily while you continue the diet. Kidney stones are formed when the acidosis in your body tends to demineralize the bones. Low pH in urine leads to the formation of certain crystals in your body, which form kidney stones.

There is evidence that using potassium citrate as a supplement helps in reducing the formation of kidney stones since that helps in reducing the level of calcium in the bloodstream. Having said that, further research is necessary to learn more about this.

Children who follow this diet to treat epilepsy often have stunted growth since the diet reduces the production of insulin, which is one of the growth factors. There is an increased risk of fracturing the bones. This arises from the altered levels of production of the insulin like growth factor 1 and acidosis. Acidosis leads to the weakening of the bones. The bones may also turn brittle which makes them sensitive.

It is always good to take a supplement of vitamins (calcium, vitamin D and multivitamins) to avoid these side effects.

Side Effects in Adults

Adults face certain complications like:

1. Weight loss
2. Constipation
3. Increased levels of cholesterol
4. Increased levels of triglycerides

Women may also develop symptoms for amenorrhea and may have certain disruptions in the menstrual cycle. We will look at how women can follow the ketogenic diet despite these side effects later in the book.

Part Two: Getting Into the Keto Mindset

How to Ease into the Ketogenic Diet

Now that you have a fair idea about this diet and its merits, let us get started. In this chapter, I have compiled several tips, which will help you get started with this diet and follow it. While this diet is easier to follow, you might still face difficulties initially, while changing your dietary habits. Patience and perseverance will have to be your best friends, when it comes to implementing any changes to your dietary habits. Therefore, I suggest you follow these tips and be patient with yourself, as you go about implementing this diet.

Buy in bulk quantities

When you are starting a new diet, obviously there will be oppositions to change. You will be tempted to eat the things that you like, irrespective of whether they are within the purview of this diet or not. The initial days are extremely tricky and will have to be dealt carefully. If you deviate in the first week itself, the chances of you coming back to this diet are pretty slim. Even if you do come back, the resolve to stick until the end might not be there. Therefore, it is important that you stay focused during the first few days. Once you get past this stage, it is only going to be easier for you to follow this diet for the rest of your life.

One suggestion to help you stay on track is to buy all your grocery items in bulk quantities. There are three key benefits of buying your groceries in bulk.

Saves money

When you buy your groceries in bulk, you save a lot of money. We all know that prices of large packets are always cheaper than average sized ones. This way, as part of staying on track, you are also saving some money. Think of this as a Costco purchase -

Saves time

Typically, you hit the grocery store at least once a week to buy your grocery items. By buying it in bulk, you are reducing the number of trips to the grocery store. We all know how going to the grocery store is such a time-consuming exercise. You can save a lot of time by reducing the number of trips to the store.

A big source of motivation

When you stock your pantry with all the essential groceries in bulk quantities, the chances of you deviating from your diet are pretty slim. You do not want to waste so many items and deviate from the diet. Although, you save a bit of money by shopping in bulk, you would definitely not want to waste the money spent on the groceries. If you are hungry, you use only the ingredients in your kitchen to cook a meal. This way, not having enough groceries is not an excuse any more for you to deviate from the diet and eat out. Therefore, having a well-stocked pantry can be a huge motivating factor, when you are trying to follow this diet.

Keep your body hydrated

When you are introducing changes to your dietary habits, it is important that you take necessary precautions. One such precaution is to keep your body hydrated at all times. Consuming enough fluids throughout the day will actually help to sustain your energy levels as well. It will also aid in the digestion process. Another advantage of drinking lots of water is that it helps in fat metabolism. Thus, you are accelerating the weight loss by keeping your body sufficiently hydrated. Make sure to drink at least 6 to 8 glasses of water every day. You can also opt for other juices, so long as they are not loaded with sugar.

These are just illustrative ground rules for your reward system. As I mentioned before, it is important that you spend some time in carefully designing your reward system, for it will help you implement the diet in an effective manner. In fact, the time that you spend upfront in designing your reward system will actually save you the time that you would end up looking for some kind of motivation to stick to the diet. If you deviate, it is going to take even more time to get back on track.

Keep a tab on the protein content

It has extremely important that you remember that this is not a high-protein diet. This is a high-fat diet and you are required to eat only just enough protein. Keep this in mind when you are buying your groceries, eating out, or preparing your meals. Make sure that the protein content in your meals is not too high. If it is indeed high, you will end up not losing any weight. When you eat too much protein, your body automatically starts secreting insulin. The rate at which your body burns the fat deposited is also affected and you will require a lot of time to lose weight. When you follow any diet and cannot see any immediate results, you will definitely be discouraged to stick to it or follow it again. Therefore, it is crucial that you do not include protein in your meals in high quantities.

Eat root vegetables in minimal quantities

While there is not much restriction on the consumption of vegetables and fruits, you really need to keep an eye on the intake of root vegetables. This is because root vegetables are loaded with sugar and carbohydrates. Since the intent of this diet is to eat carbohydrates in minimum quantities, you should keep an eye out for these vegetables. Although, I have included them in the grocery list, make sure that you buy them only in small quantities. Another thing about root vegetables is that most of them contain starch, which is just more carbohydrates. Therefore, be mindful about the inclusion of root vegetables, as part of your diet.

Find your Support Group

As I have mentioned already, the initial days of the diet are extremely tricky. You would be tempted to deviate at the first chance you get. If you are sure that you do not have a strong resolve, there is nothing wrong in taking the help of others to help you through this journey. It is important that you identify your own support group of friends and family, before you even begin this diet. A support group is one of the best ways to stick to the diet since all of you can motivate each other. When you have a support group, you no longer worry about doing what people around you are doing. You also become more confident about sticking to the diet since you have people who check your progress.

Join social groups

I have already stressed on the importance of having your own support system, before you start any diet. It is important that you get the support of your family and friends. It is equally important that you connect with other people following the same diet. This is because, when you start a diet, your body will obviously oppose it.

You might have some reactions to a certain diet, or you might have tons of questions about implementing a certain diet. Of course, you can always look it up online. It is different from getting the inputs from another person, who has successfully implemented this diet. While you can always take the help of a professional dietician, before you implement the diet, it is going to benefit you in more than one way, if you join social groups formed for people following this diet. Let us look at some of the key benefits of joining these forums.

- You can interact with different people who try to follow this diet. You can get specific feedback and inputs from them, with respect to following the diets. These insights will help you design your meal plan in such a way that you are addressing all your allergies and your preferences in the best manner possible.

- These social forums also contain suggestions for implementing this diet effectively. Each person would have shared his own success story, which could be useful, when you are trying to implement this diet. There could be specific tips, which will help you get started and follow this diet properly.

- The beauty about these social forums is that people get to share the success stories. When they receive recognition from the rest of the members, they feel motivated to keep going. As a beginner, you need every bit of motivation to hold onto this diet. When you share your success story, you will really feel good about yourself and the progress that you have made. The recognition that you get by doing so, will help you stay motivated enough to follow this diet.

- If you want to stay updated about the key findings pertaining to this diet, the best way to do so is to be part of these forums. People tend to share the latest research studies surrounding this diet and also the results of such studies. You can be abreast of all the latest studies regarding this diet and this will also reassure you that you are doing the right thing by following this diet.

- The social groups are not just for posting the good things. People often share the stories of how they deviated from the diet and what it looks for them to get back on track. These forums can provide you the opportunity of learning from others' mistakes. Therefore, when you are trying to implement this diet, you can plan your schedule and meal plan in such a way that you avoid common pitfalls.

- More than your family member or friend trying to motivate you, you would be more motivated if a person in the social group pushed you to follow this diet. This is because the person advising you is going through the same journey that makes it easier for you to relate to them. You may not relate this way with your friends or family. We tend to take the counsel of people, who have already walked the path before. Therefore, if you are thinking about deviating from this diet, these social forums can be a source of support to you.

Maintain a food journal

Getting into the habit of maintaining a food journal will actually help you in implementing any diet in an effective manner. As I said before, we do not really pay attention to what we eat, let alone worry about the harmful nature of the ingredients we are consuming. Even before you implement this diet, it is important that you learn to maintain a food journal. When you start doing this, you will be more aware about your dietary habits.

Record every meal that you consume, along with nutrition information. Now, it might not be possible to predict the nutrition value of all meals accurately, especially if you are eating them outside. So long as you put in an estimated figure, you are good to go. After recording all entries for a week, take a look at the journal. You can note down the quantity of each macro you eat every day. For instance, assess if you have been following a high carb diet, based on these entries. This information will give you an insight on what is required to implement the keto diet effectively. For example, if you are already following a high-fat and high-carb diet, you need to focus only on the reduction of the carbs intake. Maintaining a food journal will help you gain specific insights into your dietary habits and come up with a proper plan for implementing the keto diet.

The practice of maintaining a journal will also help you in sticking to the diet. For instance, if you have to record every entry in your journal, you would think twice before you deviate from the diet. When you record all your meals in a diligent manner, you can quickly catch any deviation and make sure that you compensate for it in the upcoming meals. For example, if you realize that you have consumed more carbs in your breakfast, you can skip carbs for the rest of the meals and focus only on fat and protein. This way, you are still sticking to the principles of your diet, although you should try to maintain as much consistency as possible.

Having a journal will also help you keep track of your progress. Keeping track of your progress is essential to tweak your diet plan accordingly. For instance, if you realize that you are struggling to stick to the diet, you can identify the distracting factors and come up with ways to deal with them. On the other hand, if you realize that you are making good progress, you will actually feel motivated to continue following this diet.

Stop eating out before you begin the diet

Gone are the days when we eat out only on certain occasions. Almost, all of us end up eating outside, every other day. In fact, eating home cooked meals have become such a rare thing that we do not realize what we are missing. This habit of eating out frequently could be a major dissuading factor, when you are trying to follow any diet. This is probably because the restaurants that you go to or the fast food joints that you frequent may not always have keto friendly ingredients or prepare their meals as per the principles of this diet. Even though certain dishes might look keto friendly, all the ingredients might not actually be based on the principles of this diet. In fact, if you recall, I had suggested buying sauces and flavoring agents, which do not have added sugars. There is no guarantee that these restaurants might have sourced such similar ingredients. The sauces or condiments that they use could definitely be loaded with more carbs and sugars. Therefore, it is important that you learn to reduce the number of times you eat out, before you start this diet.

I know that it is not possible to immediately bring down the number. Take it slow and do it gradually so that you are not starving. Ideally, you should be doing this at least a week before you start the diet. This way, you are preparing your body to certain dietary changes. Previously, if you were eating out 10 times a week, try to bring it down to six. As and when you go through the diet, you can bring the instances down to an even smaller number. By doing this, you are also preparing your mind for following this diet. You will be less tempted to go out and eat, when you are following the diet, if you started implementing this.

Irrespective of you start to follow any diet, this conscious decision of bringing down the number of times that you eat outside is always going to benefit you eventually. One important reason why most of us face obesity and other lifestyle related disorders is because of the drastic increase in the number of meals that we eat outside every day. Just as in the case of shopping, not all of us actually pay attention to the ingredients being used in those dishes. There are new studies emerging every other day, which keep reiterating the harmful nature of added preservatives and artificial flavoring agents. Therefore, make sure that you implement this habit, irrespective of whether you are following any diet or not.

Common mistakes to avoid

Get Salty

If you are a first-time keto dieter, you might experience few symptoms like constant headaches, fatigue, feeling feverish, etc. often referred to as keto flu. Do not worry since your body will adapt to this routine. That being said, you could prevent these symptoms. You are losing more electrolytes as you eat real, wholesome food and drink loads of water. You will need to ensure that your electrolyte levels are consistent. The easiest way to do it is by adding salt (sodium) into your body. You can mix a teaspoon of salt to your drinking water and have it once a day. You can also add sriracha or chili garlic sauce to your food as they have sodium. You can add a bit more salt while you are giving extra seasoning to your salads or other dishes. There is another benefit to consuming more salt – your body retains water effortlessly thereby reducing your trips to the restroom!

Know your WHY factor

You should always know why you are starting a new diet. You should know why you are following that diet. Do you want to follow the diet because you want to lose weight? Is it because you want to look good? Do you want to change your lifestyle? Or are you doing it to improve your health? Regardless of what the reason may be, it is important that you understand it. This is the only way you will stick to the diet. 99 percent of your diet's success lies in your mind. You need to ensure that you are mentally strong. You may want to eat some food, which will push your body out of ketosis. Ask yourself why you want to follow the ketogenic diet and use those reasons to stick to the diet.

No more snacking

Gaining better control over your appetite is one of the best things about the keto diet. You may have always given into your cravings and grabbed something to eat from the refrigerator every time you heard your stomach grumbling. You may still experience these feelings a few weeks after you begin the ketogenic diet. This is when most people give up and give into their cravings. Your body is used to specific kinds of food since you have always eaten that way. For instance, you may be used to eating something after every three hours and this habit will make it hard for you to stop yourself from walking to the refrigerator and grabbing something to eat. You need to consciously work toward switching off your mind to this habit. The best way to achieve this is by planning your meals much earlier. Meal planning or prepping plays an important role in the keto diet.

Stress management

Over-stressing yourself is going to increase the cortisol levels in your body. Cortisol is the stress hormone that increases your blood sugar level. This will make it difficult for you to lose weight. When your body experiences a consecutive rise and fall in your blood sugar levels, it sends a confusing signal to your brain. Your brain naturally assumes that it is time to refill the glycogen reserve and so it sends you a signal by telling that it needs carbs now. If you want to ensure that you lose weight on the ketogenic diet, then you need to work on your stress management.

Do not be scared of fat

It does sound silly that you need to eat more fat especially if you want to lose weight, doesn't it? If you want to lose weight and burn the excess fat in your body, you should deprive your body of carbohydrates. Carbohydrates are the primary source of energy for your body. When the body does not get enough glucose through food, it will target the glycogen. Once it completely exhausts the glycogen reserve, it begins to look for an alternate energy source. This is when your stored fat comes into the picture. Your body will target the stored body fat, burn it and break it down into fatty acids and ketones in the liver. When this happens, your body enters into the metabolic state called ketosis. So, eating more healthy fats is going to help you get rid of all the water weight and extra flab. So, fats are good here - you do not need to be scared!

Stop snacking often

Too much snacking can knock you out of ketosis as it can spike up your blood sugar levels. Since the keto diet is a low-carb, high-fat diet, stock up on high-fat food. You will be satiated when you increase your fat intake. Your appetite will decrease. If you are craving a snack, you can eat a handful of almonds. The best way to reduce too much snacking is to prepare your meals in advance so that you do not snack while you cook your meal.

Do not eat the same meal every time

It is important for you to ensure that you do not eat the same meal every day. You will get bored otherwise. There are so many keto-friendly recipes out there and all you need to do is choose the ones best for you. You can always tweak the recipes that you find on the internet to your liking. Always add some low-carb veggies to your usual keto meal and spice it up with herbs and condiments. Try to experiment with the food that you eat to make your meals interesting. This is the only way you can ensure that you stick to the ketogenic diet.

Too much protein is not good

When you eat too much protein on the ketogenic diet, your body will be pushed out of ketosis. Since you do not eat meat regularly when you follow this diet, there are times when you will overeat. Too much protein can produce glucose through the process of gluconeogenesis. Excess protein gets converted to glycogen that will then get converted to fat. Adding chicken breast to your diet routine is good but eating a whole bucket of the chicken fry is not going to do any good for your keto diet. Note down your macronutrient intake after each meal to prevent such issues.

Sleep is essential

If you are not giving your mind and body the much-required rest, your system is going to face difficulty in doing things it is supposed to do. It is important to sleep well so you can control your stress. You should give your body enough rest, so you can be energetic the following day. It is important to sleep for eight hours.

Part Three: Keto Experimenting and Tracking

Experimenting with Keto

Before you start the ketogenic diet, ensure you read everything you can about this diet. It is important to note that this diet affects people differently, and you should speak to your physician before you change your eating patterns. Start off slowly and stick to the diet for a week before you do it for a month or longer. This chapter helps you understand how to experiment with the diet. Follow the instructions below:

1. Conduct research
2. Find someone who wants to do the diet with you – a friend, family member or colleague
3. Stick to the diet for the first week
4. Try to control your cravings during the week
5. Notice how your body responds to the lack of carbohydrates
6. Continue the diet for a month
7. Observe the change and results

Try Not to Do It Alone

Find someone who wants to try this diet with you. When you try to do this alone, it becomes hard to stick to the diet.

The hardest part: Adaptation and Keto Flu

You will find yourself doing well on the first day of the diet, and you eat a healthy breakfast. The hardest part is to spend time and read labels of all the products you purchase in the supermarket. You may have done it sometimes in the past, but you find yourself looking regularly at the label. When you read labels, you realize that any food you eat contains some sugar.

At the end of the first day, you feel great. That said, you soon begin to notice some withdrawal symptoms. Extreme fatigue and sugar cravings are common symptoms. You may want to crawl into bed at 7PM every day and may not have the energy to speak to your friends or family. You may even decide to give up on the diet, and this is not a psychological feeling but a physical feeling.

This may continue for a few more days, but when your body starts to adapt to the change, you feel much better.

The Result

Well, the result was not a miracle, but you feel like it was. You wake up the following day feeling normal. You can soon resume normal activities, such as running in the morning or biking to work. When you perform these activities, you realize you are doing a better job now than you did a few months ago. You may run for a longer time or even cycle without hurting your knees, and this was not possible a few weeks ago. Since your body is used to this form of eating, you find that you are used to eating healthy and have minimal sugar cravings.

The first 30 days

Things become easy after the first 30 days, and you do not feel hungry very often since you increase your fat consumption. You learn to enjoy normal food, and do not crave for sweets and other unhealthy food. At the end of the first month, you will see that you dropped a few pounds. You lose water weight in the first month. When you overcome the first few weeks of hardship, you find that it is not difficult to stick to these eating habits. Your mind is the challenge, and you need to work on controlling your thoughts. You may eat a whole box of cookies and run around the neighborhood like a maniac to lose the extra calories you consumed.

Creativity in the kitchen

Since the main challenge is food, you become very creative. You can subscribe to numerous blogs and YouTube channels to learn different keto-friendly recipes. You may learn to bake keto friendly desserts as well. When you learn to differentiate between the different ingredients, you start creating your recipes at home.

What Benefits Can I See?

Weight loss is not the only benefit of the ketogenic diet, but the fact is you feel a lot lighter when you follow this diet. You will be more active. You may run more than you used to or even bike to work. It is important to note that the effect is not the same for everybody. Some people may need to introduce carbohydrates into their diet sooner rather than later, while they maintain their intake.

What Should You Do After Three Months?

At the end of three months, you will feel lighter, and may become too slim. You see the benefits of the diet clearly. You are –

1. More active
2. Focused
3. Less bloated
4. Thinner
5. More muscle mass

You also notice that you are conscious about the food you eat. You always read labels before you purchase anything. You may also develop some new habits, such as reducing your sugar intake, swapping complex carbohydrates with simple carbohydrates and more. You soon realize that you no longer miss all the food you craved in the past.

You only indulge occasionally and eat healthy snacks or desserts. You will be more careful about what you purchase. You also learn to differentiate between hunger and boredom.

Should You Not Have a Single Cheat Day?

Most people choose to have some cheat days in their diet, but this does not always help them. When you experiment, you may eat more carbs on some days, and some sugar, too. You may eat a few scoops of ice cream on some days or eat only grains on another, and this is absolutely fine. Do not blame or torture yourself, because you are only human, and you are bound to make mistakes. That said, try to control yourself every chance you get. Do not let one cheat day damage your progress.

What do you do Now?

The ketogenic diet transforms you in ways you cannot imagine. You may stop drinking sodas, packed fruit juices and sugar drinks because of their sugar content. You may also give up on excess sugar, and this may surprise you, especially if you are someone who loves to eat sweets. Do not worry, though, since these are good signs. You have finally learned to eat right and take care of your body.

After the first few months, your diet may change slightly. That said, you should continue to eat fewer carbohydrates, preferably simple carbohydrates. You should also read the labels carefully, so you know what food you put in your mouth. This is the easiest way to eat good quality food. You can stick to these rules only if you could follow the ketogenic diet successfully for three months. You can always choose to switch to other eating patterns while you stick to consuming keto-friendly food.

What you may have gathered by now is that your body does not necessarily need carbohydrates. You may love watermelon but stick to eating only a few slices of watermelon each time and not the whole fruit. Grains may not satiate your hunger anymore but stick to the amount you should eat. Always be considerate about the food you consume.

When you perform experiments, your dietary habits improve. You become conscious about the food you put into your mouth. You also look for healthier options. Do you think this diet is worth the try? Work on changing your habits sooner rather than later. Do you now believe it is possible to change the fuel source from carbohydrates to fats? When you conduct this experiment for three months, you find it is possible to do this. You also learn that this eating pattern is healthier and better for you. Since you conducted this experiment for more than 21 days, it is a habit now.

How to Stay on Course

Sometimes it is hard to stick to a new eating regime even if you enjoy it and know that it is good for you. We are constantly bombarded with unhealthy snacks at every street corner, supermarket and restaurant, and the accessibility to these items makes them hard to pass up. Before you start beating yourself up over that cheeseburger you had for lunch, remember that changing your eating habits is a long-term process, it takes a lot of adjustment and it is not a competition. You cannot really fail at reshaping your diet because every day provides a new opportunity for improvement.

Do not be a perfectionist

Of all the dieting pitfalls that can stop your progress in its tracks, none is as insidiously damaging as perfectionist thinking. Whether it is counting calories, obsessing about minor setbacks or trying to assemble your dinner according to a mathematical formula, it is not sustainable to have this kind of relationship with food. The drive for nourishment is one of our strongest instincts, so eating should still be about delighting your senses and making you feel full and satisfied. Follow the keto guidelines but prepare the food you would like to eat and do not be afraid to step outside your comfort zone and get inventive!

Make incremental changes

A common mistake we do when trying to lose weight is to jump right into a new eating routine, which is different from what we are used to eating. While that may work in the short term, it is rarely sustainable, and it can sometimes even cause serious health problems because it is such a shock for your body. Give yourself time to ease into the keto lifestyle by making small but meaningful changes, like giving up one carb source every couple of weeks. It is important to make sure you have given yourself ample time to adjust to the change before changing anything else. A good way to reduce transition discomfort is to add a healthy nutrient source into your diet every time you take something unhealthy out. For example, if you have decided to eliminate white flour from your diet, start replacing it with almond flour or coconut flour. This means you can continue to eat biscuits, cookies and even bread on the ketogenic diet.

Drink plenty of water

It cannot be stressed enough how important adequate water consumption is to your overall health, your sense of fullness after a meal, your energy levels, your immunity and even the way you look. Yes, water has been shown to help maintain a youthful looking skin and prevent the formation of fine lines. It is indispensable in all major bodily functions - it improves digestion, keeps the kidneys healthy, and promotes the formation of muscle tissue. Sadly, study after study has shown that most people do not drink enough water, which is a worrisome situation, especially for children. A person's water needs can vary depending on their environment and their overall health. If you are not sure how much you should be drinking, do not count on your thirst to tell you the amount of water you need. Instead, try drinking one small glass of water every hour or at least 8 tall glasses of water every day.

Surround yourself with positivity

Committing to such a life-changing journey can, at times, be stressing and overwhelming. While it is normal to feel downbeat on occasion, try not to let that become your new outlook on food. You should be looking forward to your next delicious keto dish!

Sadly, lack of support and feelings of loneliness and inadequacy are some of the most common reasons why diets, and major lifestyle changes in general, fail. If you have a source of negative emotions in your life, try dealing with that first, before making any dramatic dietary changes. We are emotional creatures, and even things that may not seem related to our dieting success can play an indirect role in shaping our motivation.

If you do not know how to infuse more positivity into your life, try doing something new. Some people like to start off their day by reflecting on a positive mantra, others prefer to engage in more social activities, travel more or pick up a light sport. Whatever you think might work for you, do not be afraid to try it, you have nothing to lose. It is also important to ensure that the people in your social circle (family, friends, even your colleagues at work) understand what you are trying to achieve and have got your back. Take your time to explain your goals to them; some of them might even want to join you on this journey.

Do not be afraid to ask for help

So, you have been on the keto diet for a couple of months now and you have been reading motivational books all week, but still cannot shake those creeping feelings of confusion and uncertainty? It is time to ask for help, may that be from your significant other, your best friend, or even a professional. Dieters often report experiencing feelings of shame and guilt for what they perceive as weaknesses or failures in conforming to a diet regime, and those feelings are far, far more dangerous than the setbacks that caused them. It is okay to make mistakes and there is no shame in admitting you need assistance in reaching your goals. Do not be afraid to talk to a certified nutritionist and you might be surprised at the insight they have to offer.

Know what to expect

If you are anxious about starting the transition to the ketogenic diet, remember that no one experience is flawless. Some people may find transitioning more difficult than others, but everyone makes mistakes and experiences setbacks at some point or another. Changing your eating habits so dramatically is no small feat, so it is wise to expect some discomfort. You are asking your body to switch energy sources that, in a way, is like switching to a different kind of battery. You may have a bit of a rocky start, feel tired often, or find it difficult to feel full after eating an entire meal. While this is normal, try not to stress your body too much.

Dial back on some of the recent changes you have made or consider new ways to substitute what you feel you have lost.

Do not neglect other aspects of your health

While dietary changes alone can make the world of a difference in improving your overall health and weight, it is immensely helpful to just be good to yourself. Things like keeping a moderately active lifestyle, getting enough sleep, taking time off work and spending it with your family, or getting a routine physical exam, will work in tandem with your new diet to help support your health and prolong your life.

If you are struggling to incorporate more physical activity into your daily routine, think simple. Walking, cycling and other outdoor activities are not only good for your body, but also for your mind and soul. Studies are now showing that even mild exercise can have a positive impact on mental health, supporting energy levels, increasing feelings of well-being and even treating depression, anxiety and stress.

Do not give up your favorite foods, turn them keto!

Thinking of any diet in terms of what you are **not** allowed to eat can quickly become frustrating and discouraging. Instead, look to keto cookbooks and the very inventive keto internet community for tips and ideas on how to turn traditional dishes into delicious keto-friendly versions. Keep in mind that going keto is not about deprivation, but about improving your diet and supporting ketosis. Because this is a high fat eating routine, you are still preserving all the deliciousness and texture of your favorite foods. In many cases, the ketogenic diet will even allow you to enhance the flavor of classic dishes by adding luscious ingredients that you might have otherwise shunned, such as heavy cream and melted butter.

Make eating healthy a lifelong goal, not a one-off project

For most people, reaching their health and weight goal is not the most difficult aspect of dieting. Keeping that weight off and making dietary changes that last a lifetime is what is truly challenging. Reaching your primary goals can happen within months, so bear in mind from the very start that you will eventually hit the maintenance phase. At this phase, you are no longer trying to shed extra weight or improve your blood test results; you are just trying to preserve what you have achieved. For long-term success, it is important that you keep making small steps and gradually work towards making the ketogenic diet your normal, everyday way of eating.

Come up with a suitable reward system

To keep you motivated to stay on track, you need to come up with your own reward system. Some of the key benefits of having a reward system in place are as follows:

- You do not have to rely on others to motivate you to stay on track. You would be motivated automatically by your own reward system and this helps you stay on track.
- When you realize that there is a reward for staying on track the entire week, you will think twice before deviating from your diet. The initial few days of dieting could be quite challenging, and you could always use some extra motivation. Having a reward system will help you with that!

However, there are certain ground rules that you need to put in place, before you design your reward system. Let us look at some of those rules. Again, these are pretty illustrative in nature. You can tweak them as you please.

Set tangible goals first

Be clear about your goals before you decide on a reward. Take some time to set your dietary goals. Do not go overboard and come up with unrealistic goals. The goals that you set should be measurable, practical and achievable. For example, you can come up with a goal of cooking all your meals for one week. Try to go for short-term goals, as they can provide you a specific sense of direction. Trust me when I say that this sense of direction will help you in implementing your diet in an effective manner.

Come up with appropriate rewards

Rewards can be quite tricky, and you need to design your reward system with care. You will have to choose the quantum of the reward, based on the effort involved. For example, if you are someone who lives on junk foods, it might be difficult for you to give it up altogether from tomorrow. Therefore, a realistic goal would be to bring down the number of days you eat junk foods from 7 to 4. You need to choose a suitable reward for the effort involved in actually cutting down the intake of junk foods by half.

If your reward is too lavish, you will be too occupied with it and lose track of the diet. On the other hand, if your reward is not sufficient, you will not be motivated to stick to the diet. Therefore, choosing the right reward is absolutely crucial, if you want to stay motivated. Do not be in a hurry. Take some time and also the help of another individual to come up with an unbiased reward system.

Time your rewards properly

If you want to derive motivation from having a reward system, it is imperative that you decide on the timing of the rewards as well. If you are trying this diet for the first time, make sure that your rewards are timely so that you do not deviate from the diet at the first opportunity that presents itself. If your reward is not immediate, you will not bother sticking to the principles of this diet. Therefore, try to reward yourself as soon as possible. At the same time, do not reward yourself in anticipation of meeting your goals. That will never do you any good.

Rewards should be in line with the diet

The whole point of having a reward system in the first place is to ensure that you follow the diet. Therefore, you should choose your rewards in such a way that it does not contradict your dieting efforts. For instance, you cannot choose a heavy carb meal as a reward for following the diet successfully for a week. Therefore, come up with healthy rewards.

Reward yourself (but not with food)

"I've been doing great keeping up with my diet this month, I think I should treat myself to a regular pepperoni pizza and a chocolate bar!" - Does this sound familiar? As tempting as this kind of reaction sounds, it is reinforcing negative ideas about your newly embraced diet. Specifically, that it is a harrowing chore you must put up with until the next time you can reward yourself with "normal" food. Thinking this way will not do you any good overall and, if you really dislike the way you are eating, you could try to improve your current diet.

That being said, it still helps to set goals and reward yourself when you achieve them, just do not do it with more food. A good way to go about it is to pamper yourself. Treat yourself to a lovely day at the spa, get a professional massage, go on a shopping spree or try an outdoor activity you have always wanted to try but never got around to. This way, you are pumping some positive reinforcement into your life and it will make you feel better about your diet.

Managing social outings

I know that it is not possible to always stay indoors and just eat home cooked meals. At some point in time, you will have to accept invitations to social outings. It is important that you stick to your diet, no matter what. While this can be tricky, it is possible. A couple of tips to help you come out of these social meetings, without deviating from your diet plan, are as follows:

Eat before you go out

If you were not sure about the menu at the meeting, it would do you good if you did not eat out much. It is not possible for you to find only keto friendly items at the dinner. Therefore, the best way to eat less out is by actually eating at home before you venture out. I know this might sound crazy but trust me you will feel good about not deviating from your diet!

Refuse the menu card

If you know which restaurant you are going to, you can actually look up the menu card online before you go out. Try to identify those items, which are based on the principles of this diet. Choose the dish that you want to eat. When you reach the restaurant, decline the menu card and order the dish that you have chosen. This way, the odds of you getting tempted by other items on the menu and ordering something, which is not permissible under your diet, are very low.

Let your host know your preference

If you are being invited to a friend or colleague's house for dinner, do let them know that you are dieting, and you would eat light. By informing them upfront, you are giving them an opportunity to have a keto-friendly dish on the menu. If that were not possible, at least you would not come across as a rude person, who keeps turning down every dish at the table. This way, you will not feel pressured to eat any dish, which is not keto friendly.

Part Four: Keto for Women

Keto for Women

Is the ketogenic diet different for women than for men? If you want an effective and fast way to lose weight, find physical and mental energy, control your sugar problem, and reduce information, the ketogenic diet is the way to go. That said, is this diet recommended for women?

This chapter explores the ketogenic diet and why it is different for women. We will also look at different tips to make the ketogenic diet work for a woman.

Why is it Difficult for Women to Lose Weight?

Let us assume that you and a friend (a man) started weight loss program together. You will stick through your caloric goals from exercise the same and maintain a diet. You look at the scale after the month; you see that the man lost more weight than you. This is not fair, but unfortunately, it is a biological process. Women have many obstacles or hurdles when it comes to losing weight. Some of these problems include:

Their Makeup

Since a woman's body constantly prepares for a pregnancy, they have at least 10% less muscle mass and more body fat stores when compared to men. Since muscles burn calories faster than fat, men have higher metabolism rate as well. This means they burn more calories when compared to women, which makes weight loss easier.

Undiagnosed PCOS

Polycystic ovary syndrome or PCOS is a common endocrine disorder. It affects close to 10% of the female population. That said, over 70% of women with this disorder are not aware of that they have it. This imbalance causes insulin resistance, irregular periods, and difficulty in maintaining an ideal body weight.

Menopause

Menopause also leads to weight gain, especially in the lower abdominal. Since women have a lower metabolism rate, the decreasing hormone levels during menopause lead to the menopause pot belly, also known as the "meno-pot."

These are some of the reasons why women have a hard time losing weight. This does not mean that the ketogenic diet cannot work for you. Research shows that the ketogenic diet is an excellent way for women to lose weight, especially if they do it right. Women can train their body to run on fats instead of carbohydrates when they switch to the ketogenic diet. This means you get to:

- To use the fat stores in your body to your advantage. When your body begins to use fat, it recognizes the cells as a source of fuel. This means you can eat fewer calories and let your body burn fat to produce energy.
- To improve your body's sensitivity to insulin. When you reduce your sugar intake, you resolve insulin resistance, PCOS and fertility issues to prevent weight loss.
- To restore or balance your hormone levels. Excess sugar and carbohydrates have significant effects on your hormonal balance. You can reset the hormone levels in your body through the ketogenic diet.

The only issue is that there is little research to help one understand the effect of the ketogenic diet. That said, let us discuss what we know so far about the ketogenic diet.

How is the Diet Different for Women?

Women must consider different aspects when it comes to their diet, and men do not have to deal with them when they choose to follow a diet.

Hormones

A change in the level of female hormones in the body affects reproduction, metabolism and stress. The levels fluctuate based on fewer carbs, menstrual cycles and lack of sleep. Men have hormones too, but female hormones are sensitive to lifestyle and dietary changes. Since the ketogenic diet is a drastic change in the diet, it becomes hard for your body to handle this change. This harms your hormones if you are not too careful.

Low Estrogen Levels

If you are in your reproduction years, you may notice a drop in the estrogen levels if you follow the ketogenic diet. When you reduce the consumption of processed food, you also reduce the consumption of soybean oil. You should ensure to maintain your estrogen levels, since low levels can lead to vaginal dryness, disruptions in your mood and sleep cycle and lower sex drive.

High Estrogen Levels

If you are nearing menopause or in it, your estrogen levels naturally decline. Experts recommend that you follow a high fat keto diet.

Increase in Cortisol

Your body produces cortisol in large quantities if there is minimal or no glucose in your body because your body cannot handle stress without glucose.

If you increase your intake of sugar, it leads to insulin resistance and increases weight.

Period

No matter what anybody says, period do suck. Women have to deal with periods and the uncomfortable symptoms every month. Why is it hard to follow the ketogenic diet during PMS?

- You crave for sweets and savory items during PMS, and this makes it hard to stick to the keto diet
- You feel like you weigh more or are bloated since you hold onto water

- It becomes difficult to digest food during PMS because of the bloating. The pain is not from your stomach and from your abdomen, so maybe you are not even hungry. You may choose to eat food that your body can digest easily
- Headaches are no joke at all, and they can compound into a keto headache if you do not watch your electrolyte and water balance
- Your cramps do not make it easier for you, and you may want to huddle on your bed with a plate of nachos, a few scoops of ice cream or a box of chocolates

Men do not have such problems, and they find it easier to stick to the ketogenic diet. Women, on the other hand, are miserable for two weeks, which makes it hard to stick to the diet.

Reducing Your Intake Quickly

Experts recommend that men should not eat too few carbohydrates when they follow the ketogenic diet. A woman, however, should never eat too few carbs. As mentioned earlier, a woman's body is sensitive to dietary changes, and a sudden decrease in carbohydrates may send your body into the starvation mode. It will hold onto your calories and not burn the fat reserves because it is starving. This shock will lead to the overproduction of different hormones like cortisol and estrogen, which can stall weight loss. When you add a few more carbs to your diet, your body learns that things are okay. It will gradually start burning the fat reserves to produce energy. You need to increase your carbohydrate intake if you are:

- Working out regularly and often perform high intensity workouts
- Active during the day
- Putting on or building lean muscle
- Unable to recover from your workouts
- Are unable to lose weight
- Pregnant
- Breastfeeding
- In the menopause or perimenopause state

We will look at different ways to control your carbohydrate intake later in this chapter. You also need to watch your caloric intake.

You May Not Eat Enough

The keto diet suppresses your appetite, and you are not always as hungry as you used to be. Since you are not hungry, you may forget to eat food. This does sound amazing, but it extremely unhealthy. You need to create a caloric deficit if you want to lose weight, but you have to give your body the calories it needs, so it can function. Do not fear fat since it helps you meet your caloric requirement. Embrace fat in the ketogenic diet. Since you cut carbs from your diet, you need to increase your fat intake, if you are:

- Pregnant
- Breastfeeding
- Burn a lot of calories during workouts
- Experience irregular periods
- Crave caffeine and sweets regularly
- Suffer from brain fog
- Prone to infections such as yeast infections, SIBO and UTIs

Breastfeeding and Pregnancy

Is it difficult for you to get pregnant? The ketogenic diet is one of the best ways to increase your chances of pregnancy. Women with PCOS have fertility issues. Their ovaries may stop ovulating, and this makes pregnancy impossible. A study was conducted on women with this syndrome, and it was found that two women who were infertile were able to conceive when they followed the ketogenic diet.

Is It Safe to Follow the Ketogenic Diet During Pregnancy?

You can follow the ketogenic diet during pregnancy. You need to speak to your gynecologist and dietician, so you get the right nutrition during pregnancy. Here are some tips to bear in mind:

- Do not try to lose weight during your pregnancy. Your baby needs all the calories and nutrients possible.
- Avoid intermittent fasting during pregnancy, since your baby will not get the required nutrition.
- Increase your carbohydrate intake to build muscles, bones and other internal structures.
- Do not reduce your caloric intake when you breastfeed, since that affects your ability to produce milk. When you eat fewer calories, the milk supply becomes less.

Mealtimes Are Tough

If you have to prepare and cook the meals at home, you may find it difficult to cook non-keto options for the rest of the family and keto meals for yourself. This is especially hard when you have children at home. When it becomes too much work to stick to the diet, you slowly lose the motivation to do it. Research shows that women view mealtimes as a way to bond with family and friends, and when they stick to their diet while people around them gorge on delicious food, they lose the will to continue with the diet.

Does this mean women cannot follow the ketogenic diet? No. Women can follow the keto diet, but they have to pace themselves.

Nailing Keto

If you do it right, the ketogenic diet can be the biggest step up for your health. The following are some tips you need to keep in mind when you choose to switch to the ketogenic diet.

Slowly Limit Your Carbs

Men can start the keto diet any day they want to and lower their carbohydrate intake from 200 grams to 25 grams. Women, however, need a little more time to adjust. Before you start the ketogenic diet, track your food intake. This process will help you manage and measure your food in macros when you follow the ketogenic diet. It also helps you identify your carb baseline. Let us assume you eat 250 grams of carbohydrates each day. You do not have to take drastic measures to shift your body into ketosis. In one study, 24 women were asked to follow a low carb diet for a span of eight weeks. Each of them lost 19 pounds and had lower insulin resistance, blood sugar levels, testosterone levels and triglycerides. This happened because they limited their carbohydrate intake to 70 grams per day. This means you do not have to jump from 250 grams to 25 grams when you start off with the diet. You should ease your body into the diet.

First Week

Try to reduce your carbohydrate intake to 150 grams per day and see if you can end the week by reducing the intake to 100 grams.

Second Week

Start with 100 grams of carbohydrates each day and end the week by reducing the intake to 50 grams.

Third Week Onwards

By the end of the third week, try to reduce your intake to 25 grams and stick to this number.

This gradual reduction helps your body adapt and adjust; however, you have to listen to your body. If you feel too tired, are hungry often or cannot finish your workout, you need to include more carbohydrates to your diet.

Switch to Intermittent Fasting

Women can lose weight easily and burn the extra fat in their body with intermittent fasting. Intermittent fasting is an eating pattern where you fluctuate between eating and fasting periods. You can fast for as long as 18 hours. The most common intermittent fasting pattern is the 16/8 method where you eat healthy meals during the eight-hour eating window and fast for 16 hours. This eating pattern gives your body the needed break from digestion.

Your body repairs itself during the fasting period. If there are no carbohydrates in your body, it will switch to the fat reserves to produce energy. This means you do not eat too many calories during the day.

Eat Healthy Food to Feed your Cravings

No woman is the same when it comes to food cravings during PMS. That said, most women crave for high calorie junk food and chocolate. Switch to one of the following keto snack items during these times. Do not succumb to your cravings and grab a bag of potato chips.

Sweet

- Chocolate Chip Keto Cookies
- Keto Brownies with Peppermint Crunch
- Keto Bars
- Chocolate Mint Keto Ice Cream
- Healthy Homemade Keto Chocolate Bars
- Keto Chocolate Mug Cake
- Chocolate Keto Chia Pudding
- Chocolate Sea Salt Peanut Butter Bites

Savory

- Creamy Keto Cauliflower Mac and Cheese
- Crispy Kale Chips
- Creamy Keto Spinach Artichoke Dip
- Keto Jalapeño Poppers
- Celeriac Everything Oven Fries

Always stay away from the scale during your period to maintain emotional and mental health. Do not ignore the gym since exercise does help to reduce the pain.

Start Resistance Training

You will not be ripped or jacked if you consciously work on building muscle. When you have more muscle mass, your metabolism improves. Your body burns more calories when you are rest and your physique will look better. Strength training also improves reproductive function and decreases belly fat, and this is no easy feat. Try to work out at least thrice a week and record your exercise routines in your journal.

Maintain a Food Journal

You need to track the food you eat, so that you meet the required macro level. You can either write it down in a journal or use a food tracking application to calculate the macros. Since your body is sensitive to changes, it is best to maintain a journal, where you write about how you feel about following the ketogenic diet. You can monitor the following in the journal:

- Cravings

- Energy levels
- Weight
- Body goals
- Exercises
- Moods and emotions
- Body measurements
- Workout recovery

You may not want to track this information, but it will help your doctor when you visit them with any issues. You can also identify the food your body cannot tolerate. The journal also helps you identify the supplements you may need for your diet.

Eat Keto-Friendly Supplements

Most women drink cranberry juice to prevent urinary tract infections since they are prone to developing it. This juice, however, is not keto friendly. Instead of avoiding cranberry juice altogether, look for a keto-friendly cranberry supplement. You can also include collagen protein if you want to improve the texture and strengthen your nails, joints, hair, and skin. This supplement also improves digestion. When you come off a cheat day or just start the ketogenic diet, eat exogenous ketones since they help your body switch easily to ketosis.

The ketogenic diet for women does take a lot more homework, and you need to pay attention to what you eat, so you get it right. This is the best decision you make for your well-being, health and appearance.

15-Day Meal Plan

Since we covered the basics of the ketogenic diet, and what you can do to stick to the diet, let us look at a 15-Day meal plan to help you start with the ketogenic diet.

Day 1

Breakfast – Breakfast Skillet

Lunch - Goat Cheese Salad with Balsamic Butter

Dinner - Bacon Cheeseburger Wraps

Day 2

Breakfast – Avocado Eggs

Lunch - White Pizza with Mushrooms and Pesto

Dinner - Cheese Meatloaf

Day 3

Breakfast – Cranberry Chocolate Chip Granola Bars

Lunch - Dill Chicken Salad

Dinner - Easy Mexican Chicken Casserole with Chipotle

Day 4

Breakfast – Cauliflower Hash Browns

Lunch - Garlic Asiago Cauliflower Rice

Dinner - Twice-Baked Spaghetti Squash

Day 5

Breakfast – Sausage Sandwich

Lunch - Chicken Bacon Saute

Dinner - Chicken al Forno with Vodka Sauce

Day 6

Breakfast – Pizza Eggs

Lunch - Buffalo Chicken Taquitos

Dinner - Baked Eggs

Day 7

Breakfast – Baked Cheese

Lunch - Goat Cheese Salad with Balsamic Butter

Dinner - Bun-less Burgers

Day 8

Breakfast – Breakfast Skillet

Lunch - Beef Soup

Dinner - Bacon Wrapped Chicken Breast

Day 9

Breakfast – Pulled Pork Breakfast Hash

Lunch - Chicken Pesto Zucchini Noodle Salad

Dinner - Bacon Cheeseburger Wraps

Day 10

Breakfast – Cinnamon Almond Butter Breakfast Shake

Lunch - Buffalo Chicken Taquitos

Dinner - Twice-Baked Spaghetti Squash

Day 11

Breakfast – Perfect Scrambled Eggs

Lunch - Lasagna Stuffed Peppers

Dinner - Halloumi Cheese with Butter-Fried Eggplant

Day 12

Breakfast – Pizza Eggs

Lunch - Tuna Stuffed Avocado

Dinner - Beef Tacos

Day 13

Breakfast – Cranberry Chocolate Chip Granola Bars

Lunch - Zoodle Alfredo with Bacon

Dinner - Zucchini Mushroom Bake

Day 14

Breakfast – Sausage Sandwich

Lunch - Garlic Asiago Cauliflower Rice

Dinner - Bun-less Burgers

Day 15

Breakfast – Perfect Scrambled Eggs

Lunch – Dill Chicken Salad

Dinner – Twice-Baked Spaghetti Sqash

Breakfast Recipes

Sausage Sandwich

Serves: 2

Ingredients:

- 2 eggs
- Salt and pepper to taste
- ¼ cup shredded, sharp cheddar cheese
- 1 teaspoon sriracha sauce or to taste
- 4 sausage patties
- 2 tablespoons cream cheese
- ½ medium avocado, peeled, pitted, sliced

Directions:

1. Follow the directions on the package and cook the sausage patties.
2. Add cream cheese and cheddar cheese into a microwave safe bowl. Cook on high in a microwave, for about 30 seconds or until it melts.
3. Add sriracha sauce to the bowl of cheese and whisk until well combined.
4. Beat eggs in a bowl with salt and pepper.

5. Place a skillet over medium flame. Add half the beaten egg. When the underside of the omelet is cooked, flip sides and cook the other side.
6. Remove the omelet and place on a plate.
7. Make the other omelet similarly.
8. Spread the cheese mixture on the omelet.
9. Place an omelet each on 2 sausage patties.
10. Cover with remaining sausage patties to complete the sandwich.
11. Serve.

Perfect Scrambled Eggs

Serves: 2

Ingredients:

- 4 large free range eggs
- 3-4 tablespoons butter
- ¾ cup single cream or full cream milk
- Salt and pepper to taste

Directions:

1. Add eggs, cream or milk, pepper and salt into a bowl and whisk lightly until well combined.
2. Place a nonstick pan over medium flame. Add butter. When butter melts, add the egg mixture. Do not stir for 20 seconds.
3. Using a wooden spoon, stir lightly. Lift and fold the egg over from the bottom of the pan.
4. Do not stir for another 10 seconds. Lift and fold the egg over from the bottom of the pan.
5. Repeat the previous step until the eggs are cooked soft overall but also runny at different spots. Turn off the heat.
6. Stir lightly and serve immediately.

Pulled Pork Breakfast Hash

Serves: 4

Ingredients:

- 4 tablespoons avocado oil
- ½ teaspoon garlic powder
- 6 Brussels sprouts, halved
- ¼ cup diced red onion
- 4 large eggs
- 2 turnips (4 ounces each), diced
- Salt and pepper
- 2 cups chopped kale, discard hard stems and ribs
- 6 ounces pulled pork
- Paprika – 1 teaspoon

Directions:

1. Place a cast iron skillet with medium-high flame. Add oil and let it heat. Add turnip, garlic powder, paprika and pepper and sauté for 3-4 minutes. Stir occasionally.
2. Stir in Brussels sprouts, onion and kale and cook until slightly tender.
3. Stir in the pork and heat thoroughly.
4. Make 4 wells at different spots in the mixture.
5. Break an egg into each cavity. Cover the pan and cook the eggs to the desired doneness.
6. Serve hot.

Breakfast Skillet

Serves: 2

Ingredients:

- ½ teaspoon oil
- ½ cup salsa
- ½ pound ground turkey
- 3 eggs

Directions:

1. Cook meat in a skillet over medium flame until it is not pink anymore.
2. Stir in the salsa and heat thoroughly. Make 3 wells in the mixture. Crack an egg into each well. Cook the eggs to the desired doneness.

Avocado Eggs

Serves: 4

Ingredient:

- 2 teaspoons olive oil
- 4 eggs, separated
- Chopped mint leaves to garnish
- 2 avocadoes, pitted, halved, scoop a little of the pulp, enough for an egg to fit in
- Salt to taste

Directions:

1. Do not discard the scooped pulp of the avocadoes.
2. Whisk together whites and salt.
3. Place a large pan with oil over medium flame. Place the avocado halves in the pan, with the cut side facing down. Cook until the cut part is light golden.
4. Turn the avocadoes, now the skin side will be down.
5. Pour the whites into the cavities of the avocadoes. It might spread on the other parts of the avocadoes. That is ok.
6. Cover the pan and cook until whites are cooked. Place a yolk in each cavity.
7. Cover and cook until the yolks are cooked to the desired doneness. Serve with scooped avocadoes.

Pizza Eggs

Serves: 2

Ingredients:

- 2 tablespoons butter
- 4 tablespoons keto friendly pizza sauce
- 4 tablespoons shredded mozzarella cheese
- Italian seasoning to taste
- 4 large eggs
- 2 tablespoons grated parmesan cheese
- 10 slices pepperoni
- Salt to taste

Directions:

1. Place a pan with butter over medium-low flame. Add butter. When butter melts, break the eggs into the pan. Do not stir.
2. When the whites are beginning to set, spread the pizza sauce over the eggs.
3. Sprinkle parmesan on top. Lower the heat and cook until whites are nearly set.
4. Sprinkle mozzarella on top. Place pepperoni slices over the mozzarella layer. Sprinkle Italian seasoning.
5. Cook until whites are fully cooked.

Cranberry Chocolate Chip Granola Bars

Serves: 8

Ingredients:

- ½ cup sliced almonds
- ½ cup flaked coconut
- ¼ cup pecan halves
- 3 tablespoons dried, unsweetened, chopped cranberries
- ¼ cup sunflower seeds
- 3 tablespoons sugar-free chocolate chips
- ¼ cup butter
- ¼ cup powdered swerve sweetener
- 1 teaspoon Yacon syrup or ½ tablespoon Sukrin gold fiber syrup
- ¼ teaspoon vanilla extract

Directions:

1. Place a sheet of parchment paper on the bottom of a small (6 x 6 inches) square baking pan such that some of the paper is hanging from the sides of the dish.
2. Place flaked coconut, pecans, almonds and sunflower seeds in the food processor bowl. Process until crumbly.
3. Remove the mixture into a mixing bowl. Add chocolate chips, cranberries and salt and stir until well combined.
4. Place a saucepan over low flame. Add butter and Yacon syrup and let it melt.

5. Add powdered swerve and whisk well. Add vanilla extract and stir. Pour into the mixing bowl. Mix well.
6. Transfer the mixture into the prepared baking pan. Press it well onto the bottom of the pan, using a flat glass or cup.
7. Bake in a preheated oven at 300° F for about 20 to 30 minutes until golden brown around the edges.
8. Let it cool completely on your countertop.
9. Cut into 8 equal portions and serve.

Cauliflower Hash Browns

Serves: 8

Ingredients:

- 2 pounds cauliflower, grated
- 1 yellow onion, grated
- 6 eggs
- Salt and pepper to taste
- 8 ounces butter, to fry

Directions:

1. Add cauliflower, onion, pepper, salt and eggs into a bowl and mix well.
2. Place a large skillet over medium flame. Add some butter. Be a bit liberal while adding butter. Allow the butter to melt.
3. Place a mound of the cauliflower mixture on the pan (1/8 of the mixture). Press with a spatula until it is about 3 to 4 inches in diameter. Make 2 – 3 hash browns or as many as can fit in the pan.
4. Cook until the underside is golden brown. Flip sides and cook the other side until golden brown.
5. Remove the hash browns with a slotted spoon and place on a plate lined with paper towels.
6. Similarly make the remaining hash browns.
7. Serve warm.

Baked Cheese

Serves: 2

Ingredients:

- 4 ounces feta cheese, cut into 2 thick slices
- Red chili flakes to taste
- 2 tablespoons thinly sliced onion
- 1 tablespoon olive oil
- 1/8 bell pepper (red), thinly sliced
- Herbal salt to taste

Directions:

1. Take 2 small baking dishes and place a slice of cheese in each. Scatter onions and bell pepper on top of the cheese.
2. Sprinkle red chili flakes and herbal salt. Drizzle oil on top.
3. Bake in a preheated oven at 400° F for about 20 minutes until the vegetables are slightly brown and cooked.

Cinnamon Almond Butter Breakfast Shake

Serves: 2

Ingredients:

- 3 cups nut milk of your choice, unsweetened
- 4 tablespoons almond butter
- 1 teaspoon ground cinnamon
- ¼ teaspoon almond extract
- Ice cubes, as required
- 2 scoops collagen peptides
- 4 tablespoons golden flax meal
- 30 drops stevia
- ¼ teaspoon salt

Directions:

1. Place all the ingredients in a blender.
2. Blitz for 30 – 40 seconds or until smooth.
3. Add collagen and pulse for 4 – 5 seconds until just combined.
4. Pour into 2 glasses and serve.

Lunch Recipes

Goat Cheese Salad with Balsamic Butter

Serves: 4

Ingredients:

- 20 ounces goat cheese
- 4 ounces butter
- 6 ounces baby spinach
- ½ cup pumpkin seeds
- 2 tablespoons balsamic vinegar

Directions:

1. Place goat cheese slices in a baking dish that has been greased with cooking spray.
2. Bake in a preheated oven at 400° F for 10 minutes.
3. Place a pan with pumpkin seeds over medium-high flame. Keep stirring until light golden and the seeds are popping.
4. Reduce the heat to low heat. Stir in the butter and cook until pumpkin seeds are golden brown.
5. Stir in the vinegar and simmer for 2 – 3 minutes.
6. Remove from heat.
7. Divide spinach among 4 serving plates. Divide the cheese among the plates.
8. Drizzle balsamic butter on top and serve.

Beef Soup

Serves: 4

Ingredients:

- ½ pound ground beef
- 2 cups beef bone broth or chicken broth
- 6 tablespoons keto ranch dressing
- 1 ½ tablespoons taco seasoning, divided
- 1 can (14.5 ounces) diced tomatoes with its liquid

To garnish: Optional

- A handful fresh cilantro, chopped
- Shredded cheddar cheese

Directions:

1. Place a soup pot with beef over medium-high flame. Cook until it is not pink anymore.
2. Discard released fat if required.
3. Stir in a tablespoon of taco seasoning and half the broth. Cook until the mixture is nearly dry.
4. Stir in rest of the broth. Add tomatoes and ½ tablespoon taco seasoning and mix well.
5. Let it cook for 4 – 5 minutes. Stir frequently.
6. Turn off the heat. Let it rest for a couple of minutes. Add ranch dressing and stir.
7. Divide into soup bowls. Sprinkle cheddar cheese and cilantro on top and serve.

White Pizza with Mushrooms and Pesto

Serves: 4

Ingredients:

For crust:

- 4 eggs
- 1 ½ cups almond flour
- 2 teaspoons baking powder
- 1 cup mayonnaise
- 2 tablespoons ground psyllium husk powder
- 1 teaspoon salt

For topping:

- 4 ounces mushrooms, sliced
- 4 tablespoons olive oil
- 6 ounces shredded cheese
- 2 tablespoons green pesto
- Salt to taste
- 1 cup sour cream or crème fraiche
- Pepper to taste

Directions:

1. To make crust: Add eggs and mayonnaise into a bowl and whisk well. Add the rest of the ingredients for the crust and mix well.
2. Let the dough rest for 5 minutes.

3. Place a sheet of parchment paper on a baking sheet. Place the dough on it.
4. Grease a rolling pin with some oil and roll the dough into a circle of about ½ inch thickness.
5. Bake in a preheated oven at 350° F bake for about 10 – 15 minutes or until light brown.
6. Let the crust cool for 10 minutes.
7. Invert the crust on a cooling rack and peel off the parchment paper.
8. Add mushrooms, pesto and olive oil into a bowl and mix well. Add salt and pepper to taste and mix again.
9. Pour the sour cream on the crust and spread it evenly. Sprinkle cheese over the crust. Spread the mushroom mixture over the cheese layer.
10. Bake for 8 – 10 minutes or until the cheese melts.
11. Cut into 4 equal wedges and serve with a salad of your choice if desired.

Tuna Stuffed Avocado

Serves: 2

Ingredients:

- 2 cans (5 ounces each) packed tuna, drained
- ½ teaspoon dried dill
- 2 medium avocadoes, halved, pitted
- 4 tablespoons keto friendly mayonnaise or Greek yogurt
- Salt and pepper to taste

Directions:

1. Add tuna, dill, salt, pepper and mayonnaise into a bowl and stir.
2. Stuff this mixture into the avocado halves and serve.

Lasagna Stuffed Peppers

Serves: 2

Ingredients:

- 1 large sweet peppers, halved, deseeded
- 6 ounces ground turkey
- ½ cup shredded mozzarella cheese
- ½ teaspoon garlic salt, divided
- 6 tablespoons crumbled ricotta cheese,

Directions:

1. Season peppers with ¼ teaspoon garlic salt. Place them in a baking dish.
2. Divide turkey equally and stuff it inside the bell pepper halves. Press it well.
3. Bake in a preheated oven at 400° F for about 30 minutes.
4. Divide the ricotta and spread over the turkey. Season with remaining garlic salt.
5. Sprinkle 2 tablespoons mozzarella cheese on top of each bell pepper half.
6. Bake for 30 minutes or until the top is golden brown.

Dill Chicken Salad

Serves: 4

Ingredients:

- ½ pound chicken breast, cooked, cubed
- 3 tablespoons finely chopped onions
- ¾ tablespoon Dijon mustard
- Salt and pepper to taste
- ¼ cup diced celery
- 6 tablespoons keto friendly mayonnaise
- 1 ½ tablespoons chopped fresh dill or 1 teaspoon dried dill
- Lettuce leaves to serve

Directions:

1. Add all the ingredients into a bowl and stir.
2. Place lettuce leaves on a serving platter. Divide the salad among the lettuce leaves and serve.

Zoodle Alfredo with Bacon

Serves: 2

Ingredients:

- 4 ounces bacon, chopped
- 1 clove garlic, minced
- ¾ cup heavy cream
- ½ pound zucchini, trimmed
- Salt and freshly ground pepper to taste
- ½ shallot, chopped
- 2 tablespoons white wine
- ¼ cup grated parmesan cheese+ extra to garnish

Directions:

1. Cook bacon in a pan, over medium flame until crisp. Remove with a slotted spoon and place on layers of paper towels.
2. Retain about a tablespoon of bacon drippings and discard the rest.
3. Add shallot into the pan and cook for a couple of minutes.
4. Insert the garlic while stirring and cook for a few seconds, until aromatic. Pour wine and simmer until it is half its original quantity.
5. Meanwhile, make noodles of the zucchini using a spiralizer or julienne peeler.
6. Pour cream and simmer on low heat. Add parmesan and simmer until slightly thick.

7. Stir in the zucchini noodles. Heat thoroughly. Add bacon and stir. Serve hot.

Garlic Asiago Cauliflower Rice

Serves: 3

Ingredients:

- 1 small head cauliflower, grated to rice like texture (About 4 cups after grating)
- ½ tablespoon extra-virgin olive oil
- ¼ cup finely grated Asiago cheese
- 1 tablespoon unsalted butter
- 1 teaspoon garlic herb seasoning blend

Directions:

1. Place a heavy skillet over medium-high flame. Add oil and butter. When butter melts, add seasoning blend and cauliflower and mix well.
2. Stir occasionally and cook until cauliflower is tender but not mushy.
3. Stir in the cheese and serve.

Chicken Bacon Saute

Serves: 4

Ingredients:

- 2 chicken breasts, cut into small cubes
- 2 tablespoons garlic powder
- Salt to taste
- 8 slices bacon, diced
- 4 tablespoons Italian seasoning
- 2 tablespoons avocado oil

Directions:

1. Place a pan with oil over medium flame. When oil is heated, add chicken and bacon and stir.
2. Once the chicken and bacon is cooked thoroughly, add garlic powder, salt and Italian seasoning and mix well.
3. Serve hot.

Chicken Pesto Zucchini Noodle Salad

Serves: 2

Ingredients:

- ½ pound chicken breasts, cooked, shredded
- 2.5 ounces cherry tomatoes, halved
- 1 medium zucchini, trimmed
- 4 ounces sugar-free green pesto
- 2 ounces feta cheese, crumbled
- ½ tablespoon olive oil, to drizzle on top

Directions:

1. Make noodles of the zucchini using a spiralizer.
2. Add zucchini noodles and pesto into a bowl. Toss until zucchini is well coated with pesto.
3. Add tomatoes, chicken and feta and toss lightly.
4. Trickle olive oil on top and serve.

Buffalo Chicken Taquitos

Serves: 4

Ingredients:

- 12 slices mozzarella cheese
- 4 tablespoons buffalo sauce to serve
- 3 cups cooked or grilled, shredded chicken
- Keto friendly ranch dressing (optional)

Directions:

1. Place a silicone baking mat on a baking sheet. Lay the cheese slices on the mat.
2. Bake in a preheated oven at 350° F for about 8 minutes or until the edges on the outside are crispy and brown.
3. Take out the baking sheet from the oven and let it cool for a couple of minutes.
4. Spread chicken on one of the edges of the cheese slice. Roll the cheese slices along with the filling and place on a serving platter, with the seam side facing down.
5. Serve along with ranch dressing and buffalo sauce.

Dinner Recipes

Bun-less Burgers

Serves: 6

Ingredients:

<u>For burgers:</u>

- 2 pounds ground beef
- 2 tablespoons Mc Cromicks Montreal Steak Seasoning
- 2 tablespoons Worcestershire sauce
- Salt and pepper to taste
- Oil, to grease, as required

<u>For caramelized onions:</u> Optional

- 8 ounces sliced onions
- 4 tablespoons bacon drippings or olive oil
- 1 teaspoon erythritol

Directions:

1. To make burgers: Add beef, steak seasoning and Worcestershire sauce into a bowl and mix well, breaking the meat simultaneously as you mix in.
2. Divide the mixture into 6 equal portions and shape into patties. Make a dent in the center of each patty.
3. Preheat the grill. Grease the grill grate by brushing with oil.

4. Sprinkle salt and pepper all over the patties and place on the heated grill. Grill the burgers to the way you prefer it cooked. Flip the burgers a couple of times while grilling.
5. To make caramelized onions: Place a nonstick pan with oil over medium-low flame. Add onions and stir. Cook until translucent.
6. Add erythritol and stir. Cook until golden brown, stirring occasionally.
7. Divide equally the onions and spread over the burgers.

Cheese Meatloaf

Serves: 12

Ingredients:

- 2.2 pounds minced meat
- Salt and pepper to taste
- 4 buffalo mozzarellas
- 2 tablespoons dried marjoram
- 4 eggs
- 4 leeks

Directions:

1. Chop the white part of the leeks into smaller pieces. Separate the individual leaves of greens of the leeks. You may need to use more leek leaves.
2. Place a pot of water over high heat and bring to a boil. Turn off the heat.
3. Drop the leek leaves into the pot. Let the leaves remain in the pot for 3 to 4 minutes.
4. Drain off the water and immerse in cold water for a minute. Drain and set aside.
5. Add meat, whites of leeks, marjoram, eggs, pepper and salt into a bowl and mix well.
6. Take a large loaf pan (use 2 smaller ones if you do not have a large one) and cover the bottom of the pan with the leek leaves such that the leaves are on the sides of the loaf pan as well.
7. Place half the meat mixture on the bottom as well as the sides of the pan. Press it well to adhere.
8. Place the mozzarella cheese in the loaf pan. Cover the cheese with remaining meat mixture.
9. Place leek leaves on top of the meat as well. The meat should be well covered with the leek leaves. Cover the loaf pan with aluminum foil.
10. Bake in a preheated oven at 350° F for about 50 minutes. Uncover and bake for 10 minutes.
11. Cool for 30 – 40 minutes before slicing and serving.

Bacon Cheeseburger Wraps

Serves: 2 (3 wraps each)

Ingredients:

- 3.50ounces bacon
- ¾ pound ground beef
- 6 iceberg lettuce leaves
- 2 ounces cheddar cheese, shredded
- 2 ounces mushrooms, sliced
- Salt and pepper to taste

Directions:

1. Place a skillet with bacon over medium flame. Cook until crisp.
2. Remove bacon with a slotted spoon and place on a plate lined with paper towels. Do not discard the fat from the pan.
3. When bacon is cool enough to handle, crumble or chop the bacon into smaller pieces.
4. Add mushrooms into the same pan and cook until brown. Remove mushrooms from the pan and place with the bacon.
5. Add beef into the same pan. Sprinkle salt and pepper and mix well. Cook until meat is cooked. Break it simultaneously as it cooks. Turn off the heat.
6. Place the lettuce leaves on a serving platter. Divide the meat among the lettuce leaves.

7. Divide equally the bacon and mushrooms, and scatter over the meat. Scatter cheddar cheese on top. Wrap the lettuce leaves over the filling and place with its seam side facing down.
8. Serve.

Easy Mexican Chicken Casserole with Chipotle

Serves: 4

Ingredients:

- 1 ½ cups cooked, shredded chicken
- 8 ounces salsa
- Ground chipotle pepper to taste
- 4 ounces cream cheese, softened
- 4 ounces shredded cheddar cheese

Directions:

1. Set aside half the cheddar cheese and add rest of the ingredients into a greased baking dish. Mix well.
2. Sprinkle remaining cheese on top. Garnish with some more chipotle pepper.
3. Bake in a preheated oven at 400° F for about 20 minutes. Until the cheese melts and is bubbling.

Chicken al Forno with Vodka Sauce

Serves: 3

Ingredients:

- 1 pound chicken breast, cooked, chopped into bite size pieces
- ¼ cup grated parmesan cheese
- ¾ cup keto friendly vodka sauce
- Baby spinach to serve, as required (optional)
- 8 ounces fresh mozzarella cheese

Directions:

1. Grease a baking dish with some oil. Spread chicken in the dish.
2. Drizzle vodka sauce over the chicken. Scatter parmesan cheese and mozzarella on top.
3. Bake in a preheated oven at 400° F for about 20 to 30 minutes or until the mixture is heated thoroughly and is bubbling.
4. Serve over baby spinach if desired.

Bacon Wrapped Chicken Breast

Serves: 3

Ingredients:

- 3 chicken breasts, halved widthwise, cut into thin pieces
- ¼ pound bacon, halved
- Sugar-free BBQ sauce to serve
- 1 tablespoon seasoning rub
- 2 ounces shredded cheddar cheese

Directions:

1. Grease a rimmed baking sheet with some cooking spray.
2. Sprinkle seasoning rub over the chicken and rub it well into it.
3. Place chicken on the baking dish. Place a piece of bacon on each of the chicken slices.
4. Place baking sheet on the top rack in the oven.
5. Bake in a preheated oven at 400° F for about 20 to 30 minutes or until bacon is crisp.
6. Scatter cheese on top of the bacon and continue baking for another 10 minutes or until cheese is bubbling and is golden brown at a few spots.
7. Serve with BBQ sauce.

Baked Eggs

Serves: 2

Ingredients:

- 6 ounces ground meat (lamb or beef or pork)
- 4 ounces shredded cheese
- 4 eggs
- Salt and pepper to taste

Directions:

1. Add ground meat, salt and pepper into a baking dish and mix well. Spread the meat evenly.
2. Make 4 wells in the mixture. Crack an egg into each well. Sprinkle salt and pepper over the eggs.
3. Scatter cheese on top.
4. Bake in a preheated oven at 400° F for about 15 minutes or until the eggs are cooked.

Zucchini Mushroom Bake

Serves: 2

Ingredients:

- 1 ½ cups sliced fresh mushrooms
- 1 ½ cups sliced zucchini
- ½ onion, sliced
- Salt to taste
- ¼ teaspoon dried basil
- ¼ cup shredded cheddar cheese

Directions:

1. Add all the ingredients except cheese into a greased baking dish. Toss well.
2. Spread it evenly. Cover the dish with foil.
3. Bake in a preheated oven at 350° F for about 30 minutes or until vegetables are cooked.
4. Scatter cheese on top and bake without covering, until cheese melts and is bubbling.

Halloumi Cheese with Butter-Fried Eggplant

Serves: 4

Ingredients:

- 2 eggplant, halved lengthwise, cut into ½ inch thick slices
- 20 ounces halloumi cheese
- Salt and pepper to taste
- 6 ounces butter
- 20 black olives
- 1 cup keto friendly mayonnaise

Directions:

1. Place a large skillet over medium-high flame. Add butter. Allow the butter to melt.
2. Place cheese on one end of the pan and eggplant slices on the other end of the pan. Cook the eggplants and cheese. Turn the cheese and eggplants when the underside is golden brown. Cook the other side until golden brown.
3. Serve cheese and eggplant with olives.

Twice-Baked Spaghetti Squash

Serves: 4

Ingredients:

- 2 medium spaghetti squash, halved lengthwise, deseeded
- 2 cups shredded mozzarella cheese
- Chopped fresh garlic leaves or basil leaves, to garnish (optional)
- 2 cups keto friendly pasta sauce
- Salt and pepper to taste

Directions:

1. Place spaghetti squash on a baking sheet, with the cut side facing down.
2. Bake in a preheated oven at 375° F for about 45 minutes or until the spaghetti squash is cooked.
3. When the squash is cool enough to handle, shred the squash with a pair of forks. Retain the shells of the squash.
4. Add shredded squash into a bowl. Add pasta sauce and mix well. Fill the mixture into the squash shells. Place the shells on the baking sheet.
5. Top with mozzarella cheese.
6. Place the baking back in the oven and bake until cheese melts and is bubbling.
7. Serve along with the shells.

Beef Tacos

Serves: 2

Ingredients:

- ½ pound ground beef
- ½ can Rotel tomatoes with green chilies
- Taco seasoning to taste

To serve:

- Lettuce leaves or keto friendly tortillas or taco shells.

Directions:

1. Place a skillet over medium flame. Add beef and cook until it is not pink anymore.
2. Add tomatoes and taco seasoning and mix well.
3. Cover and cook until meat is cooked through. Stir often.
4. Serve over lettuce leaves or tortillas or in taco shells.

Conclusion

Thank you for purchasing the book.

If you want to follow the ketogenic diet, and you do not know where to start, you have come to the right place. This book contains all the information you need about the ketogenic diet. You will also come across a few tips that you can use to make it easier for you to follow this diet.

It is difficult for people to follow the ketogenic diet, since there are many food groups they should avoid. This book leaves you with some tips to help you ease into this diet, and also leave you with some strategies to help you continue to follow this diet. Since the ketogenic diet is difficult for women to follow, the book also sheds some light on why this is the case and some tips to help you overcome these difficulties. The book also provides information on how you should ease into the diet, and what you should do to continue to follow the diet.

I hope you find the information in the book helpful and wish you luck on your journey.

Resources

https://www.ketodietyum.com/keto-diet-plan/

https://medium.com/wolff-experiments/3-months-of-keto-9aaa37e5950c

https://perfectketo.com/keto-for-women/

https://www.healthline.com/nutrition/7-tips-to-get-into-ketosis#section7

https://www.healthline.com/nutrition/10-benefits-of-low-carb-ketogenic-diets#section10

https://www.everydayhealth.com/diet-nutrition/ketogenic-diet/steps-beginners-should-take-before-trying-keto-diet/

https://medium.com/@JPMcCarter/the-top-12-keto-myths-debunked-after-150-000-days-of-patient-care-9502383d4e8c

https://www.healthline.com/nutrition/9-myths-about-low-carb-diets#section10

https://www.eatright.org/health/weight-loss/fad-diets/what-is-the-ketogenic-diet

https://www.muscleandfitness.com/nutrition/gain-mass/science-behind-ketogenic-diet/

https://ketofatfurnace.com/10-ways-to-stay-motivated-on-the-keto-diet/

https://www.everydayhealth.com/ketogenic-diet/diet/keto-diet-myths-you-shouldnt-believe/

https://ninateicholz.com/ketogenic-diet-myths-vs-facts/

9 781922 462053